An imprint of
Beautifully Designed For More
357 N. Houston Street
Maryville, TN 37801
www.beautifullydesignedformore.com

First Published in the United States of America 2021
By IngramSpark
This edition published in 2021
Text copyright © Whitney Carrión 2021
www.whitneycarrion.com
Illustrations copyright © Wavelet Designs LLC 2021
www.waveletdesigns.com

Whitney Carrión and Wavelet Designs have asserted their rights to be identified as the author and illustrator of this work under the Copyright, Designs and Patents Act 1988

All rights reserved | ISBN 978-1-7363277-1-5

Printed in the USA

Editor: Aimee Larsen www.aimeelarsen.com
Photography: Ryan Lee Photography www.rlpsavannah.com

# How to Be A Watchdog For Our Youth

by Whitney Carrión

Special Acknowledgement to Professor Jeanie Thies

# Table of Contents:

**Part 1: Why & How........................1**

**Part 2: Out & About....................13**

**Part 3: Education........................23**

**Conclusion....................................44**

**Acknowledgements.....................46**

**Jeanie Thies Biography................53**

**Acknowledgements Con't..........58**

**About the Author.........................49**

# Part 1: Why & How

**Why I Wrote This Book:**
Parents, in this book, you'll have a plethora of tips, advice, warning signs, and action steps to take, to ensure you and your child(ren) are least likely to be susceptible to any sort of sexual assault, attack, or human trafficking. There is a big emphasis in this book on protecting your children from pedophiles and human traffickers. However, being equipped with this knowledge could also help prevent a physical attack/abduction on you and/or your children. Also, I know I direct a lot of my content toward parents, but this book will help equip and inform any adult who is ever and will ever be put in charge of caring for children. Just think of all those people who fill these roles: doctors, lawyers, teachers, camp counselors, youth pastors, babysitters, siblings, cousins, grandparents, youth sports coaches, etc.

Basically, if you plan on being in charge of a child's well-being at any point in your life, this book is for you, or a great gift for anyone in the roles above.

I also want to invite you to join the "Watchdog Brotherhood," where our motto is:
*If you see something, say something.*
You can go to my website, www.whitneycarrion.com, and purchase a Watchdog bracelet. This is a great reminder to be a voice for all children.

You can also visit my website to learn more about our nonprofit organization, Bunchabighearts for Africa, which rescues and rehabilitates trafficking victims, in Jesus' name.

Not only will I equip you to lead a safer life with your family, but I also want to equip you with some signs to look out for just in case you happen to encounter someone in public who may be a victim of abuse or who is currently being trafficked. Believe it or not, you probably have before and you just didn't know the signs. Knowledge is power and can be the single best defense you have against these crimes. Knowing what to look for just may be the best chance at rescuing another victim out of trafficking.

**My Law Enforcement Background:**
I studied criminal justice with a pre-law and juvenile justice concentration. When I say I studied it, I mean thoroughly; I lived and breathed it and became very passionate about it. I wrote my senior paper on "The treatment of Pedophiles," and that's when I was horrified to learn that there was no formal rehabilitation nor treatment program for pedophilia; just incarceration and release. Which always stuck with me.

When I graduated in 2009, I actually tested for a few years with police departments in the tri-state area, (Wisconsin, Illinois, Missouri, Indiana...etc). The process to get hired onto a police force is very rigorous. The process can be intense and you may not even get a call back (if at all) for several months or even a few years. So, I was testing as many weekends as I could, to try and get in front of as many police departments as possible.

I was eventually offered a job with a Police Department in the Chicago-land area. I say, "eventually" because this was during the recession when over 20,000 officers in the state of Illinois alone had been laid off.

At that time, if anyone was getting hired on at departments, it was usually formerly laid-off officers. So, I never wound up with a formal career in my field of study. By the time I was offered a position, it was a few years after testing, and I was already in a new season of life and deeply embedded into a 2-year career in the health and fitness industry. Soon after that, I became a military wife, and the constant moving around didn't allow for any type of conventional "brick and mortar career."

Even though my career wasn't in law enforcement, my training, and passion to advocate and protect people increased when I became a mother. This is one of many reasons why I wrote this children's book and handbook.

## Who Am I To Be Teaching On This?

I can answer that simply: as a parent myself, I care enough about the welfare of your children to do so. Periodt.

I prayed for years for the Lord to bring me a cause that I was passionate enough about, to DO something. Seems funny right? As a follower of the Lord, Jesus Christ, I am compelled to give back to those that are less fortunate. I've been a dutiful giver to many causes. While almost all "causes" pull on my heartstrings, none of them so passionately wreck me to a point where I often stay up late at night stewing over it, until this one.

I spent four years studying criminal & juvenile justice and caught a fire for doing my part to help keep my community safe. It just never settled with me that the most vulnerable beings on God's green Earth could be made targets of such heinous crimes. However, because many activists worked hard to catch our attention and shed light on this gruesome crime in the beginning months of 2020, I guess you could say I became, "WOKE."

I decided it was time to do my part and use the education that my parents', Sallie Mae, and my water polo scholarship had paid for, many years ago. While I am only one person, I know that sometimes it just takes ONE VOICE to shake people loose of that monotonous trance we can often find ourselves in while going about our day-to-day lives.

I pray if needed, this advice just might save your life one day too. In fact, my hope is that you never have to find out if it does; but should that dire situation ever come up, I also pray you find yourself well equipped.

So today my friends, I have come to be that voice of reason. I have come to DISRUPT, to shake loose, to awaken, to equip, to educate, to empower, and to ARM YOU with the best that I have. All in order to prevent further crimes of this nature from happening. This book will serve as the truth until every child is returned home, and until every vulnerable human is once again safeguarded.

If you're ready for such a mission, read on, my fellow vigilantes.....

## Let's Start with Some Facts:

Right out of the gate, I want to squash a common misconception about trafficking and that is: *having male children does not exempt your family from the possibility of being targeted.*

There's just as big of a "need to fulfill" in that dark world, for adolescent boys, as there is for adolescent females. In fact, of all sex crimes, the highest repeat sex offenses are those crimes committed by adult males on adolescent males.

Another shocking statistic to note, that when it comes to these offenders, they are more likely to be someone the victim knows, likes, and trusts, versus a random attacker. This is a scary fact that I will dive into more later. For now, let's focus on the facts and educate you on what you need to know when you're in public with your child beginning with...

**Human Trafficking** is known as modern-day slavery that involves force, fraud, or coercion to obtain some type of labor or commercial sex act (DHS.gov).

Human trafficking isn't just about sexual abuse; perhaps even more horrifying is it can also be about organ harvesting on the black market, and old-fashioned slave labor as well. Sexual exploitation is the most common type of human trafficking as it accounts for 79% of the trade (unodc.org).

- The economic sectors that profit most from human trafficking are agriculture, domestic work, restaurants, manufacturing, entertainment, hospitality, and the commercial sex industry.

So, when you think about the number of times you ate at a restaurant and didn't pay attention to the boy bussing your table, when you were at a hotel and you didn't even look at the maid offering you towels, or when you visited that local farmer's pumpkin patch with your kids during Fall time......could any of those workers have been slaves? It's a chilling thought, right? It makes me CRINGE. This book isn't meant to serve as another reason for us to beat ourselves up over our not knowing; we already do that enough. So, don't do that. Let's just agree to take this education going forward to do better and BE BETTER because of it, yeah?

As soon as I began to dive deeper into this topic, it reaffirmed over and over, that modern-day slavery still exists; it's happening right under our noses. The best way I KNOW how to do my part to put an end to this sick trade is to educate, equip, and empower as many parents as I can about its existence and the ways in which we can lessen our chances of being targets.

## Disclaimer Going Forward:

*These tips are not and could never be ALL the tips and warnings you should heed; the slave trade is sadly ever-evolving and ever-growing. Thus, so are the "luring tactics" that the professionals use to capture our children. However, I will be illustrating some of the "not so obvious" warning signs to look out for and action steps to take in order to make yourselves and your children less susceptible to harm.*

## Protect Yourself, Protect Your Family:

If you believe in carrying weapons, you should. Something as simple as a quick maneuver of having your keys woven through your fingertips of one hand and your other hand around your child will make you/child less susceptible to an attack.

When my husband was deployed for a year, and I was on my own with my 1-year-old daughter all the time, a family friend gave me a neat tool called the "kitty cat defense keychain." Looks just like a key chain, but fits like brass knuckles, and has two "kitty cat ears" formed into spikes and the whole thing was made out of a very strong resin material. It was cheap too! Less than $10. I'd walk in and out of the parking lots with my baby on one hip, and the kitty cat on the knuckles of my other hand.

*There are many self-defense tools one can obtain online; you'll just want to check your state's laws on such weapons of defense and find one that's right for you if you feel you need such a tool. Laws are changing every day. Texas is an example with their House Bill 446 making the kitty ears illegal in Texas. Know your rights.*

I know we all have different beliefs on guns and weapons, but I'm not here to debate. The truth of the matter is, I hope you NEVER have to need or use a tool, spray, or weapon. I DON'T ever want to be put in a position where I'm forced to protect my family without a way to do so either! I can't even imagine. For the sake of being vigilant, it is of my strong opinion that we all MUST IMAGINE exactly that for the moment. In the name of protection, it is our duty to protect our children and ourselves. In the event that you ARE attacked, I bet you'll be wishing you had more than just your bare hands to defend your most precious babies and your own body with, RIGHT?

We've all seen videos of children quite literally being wrestled out of a parent's arms, or taken right out of a grocery cart, or attacked right out on the patio of an outdoor restaurant. Having some sort of defense will absolutely deter an attack. Know that a predator will only strike if they think they can physically outrun or overpower you.

Any reason you can give them to believe differently is a good idea. In fact, most of these crimes we are discussing aren't even really about sex, to begin with; they're about power and a very successful economic venture. There is no end to the thirst in this dark underground world, therefore trafficking is an extremely lucrative business.

These criminals get gratification from overpowering another human being; hence the vulnerable targets at hand.

Boils your blood right?

I feel you, mine too. That is why I'm writing this.

Believe it or not, something as small as even making steady eye contact with every passerby and/or suspicious person can be enough to deter a criminal in many instances. This is because most predators would rather catch you (the parent or protector) off guard. Sometimes just staring them down with that parental "NOT TA'DAY, BUDDY" look can be enough to signal to them that you are NOT the victim they are looking for. #YesMamaBear

You also want to ensure any other caretaker in your home is equipped too. I took the time to educate my nanny who was with my now 2 and 5-year-old daughter eight hours a day in this season. Even though we live on a military base and I'm home with all of them, she does take them to the park and does run errands and do fun little day trips with them. She's armed, vigilant, and she's never afraid to draw her weapon when needed and she has before!

Thank goodness she was prepared.

# Part 2: Out & About

**Leaving Home:**

We're going to start with some tips to note when leaving your home.

This isn't me trying to create a phobia for you in leaving your house. But there are some steps you can take for positive reassurance and to be proactive.

First, you don't want to be juggling too many things while walking with your child in public. As in, you don't want to be carrying too many objects and you definitely don't want to be distracted on the phone, fidgeting with a seatbelt, carrying a ton of bags, having your back to your child, etc.

Second, it's always good to have your child within an arms-length of you or holding your hand, no matter their age. The best rule of thumb when leaving the house and having to load up a bunch of stuff is to leave your child inside the home and then secure all your items in your car. After that is completed, your children exit the home at the same time you do, and they're never more than an arms-length away from you.

Children can be abducted in broad daylight in our own yards. An example of this is the Jaycee Dugard story. She was held captive for 18 years and was literally taken out of her family's front yard; her stepdad saw it happening from inside their house and tried to chase the perpetrator down, but was unsuccessful.

Some of these professional traffickers are so well trained, not just in the retrieval of a human, but in the getaway plan, that police and federal agents are quite often thwarted. So, our goal here is to prevent you from ever having to be in that situation from the start.

## While Shopping With Your Child(ren):

If you're in a public place, like a grocery store or mall parking lot, pushing your cart while your kiddos walk near you, these are the steps I encourage you to take.

1. Ensure each child is within an arms-length of you.
2. Ensure they walk on the inside of you and you're on the outside. Meaning, you put yourself between your child and the crowd; your child walks on the inside closest to the wall (when inside) or immobile objects (like a row of cars and you on the outside).
3. Unlock the car, and have both children get in on the same side of the car so that you are standing in between them and the car.
4. While buckling one, have the keys and purse on the floor of the car in front of you and keep the groceries in the cart. I'd rather someone steal that than my children, so my priority is my children. Always watch the older kids buckle themselves.
5. Close both doors and lock the car.*
6. Go around back and open the trunk and load groceries in the car. All while keeping an eye on your surroundings.

7. Then close the groceries in the trunk and lock the car again.

8. Push your cart to the buggy garage while keeping an eye on your locked car with the keys and any weapon you have.**

9. Walk back into the car, unlock it. Get in. Lock again.

10. Then do not hesitate in leaving.

*When it's hot out, I ensure my car is started while the kids are buckled inside with full-blown AC on. I am able to still lock my car with my key fob and I can quickly return my cart back to the buggy garage. If that isn't an option, it is a good idea to crack windows when kids are left in a car for any amount of time.*

**park as close as possible to a cart return/ buggy garage.*

*If someone trusted is with me, I have them load the groceries & handle returning the grocery cart, while I load the children up and secure them.*

## Beauty Tips You May Want to Consider:

I remember my Victimology professor telling us that when we wear our hair in a ponytail, it makes us an easier target. A predator can quickly grab a whole head's worth of hair from one quick snatch of our ponytail and thus, very easily overpower us. Whereas, if we have our hair down, it's harder for them to get a good hold on a majority of our hair, and we could more easily fight them off, as we'd have more control of our head.

My sister was actually attacked once. The guy came behind her while she was trying to open up the door to her apartment complex. He was able to drag her from the stoop to his car because he was able to easily get a whole grip full of her hair because it was secured in a ponytail. She wound up fighting him off once he got her to his car because she thought quickly. If her hair had been down and she had been more aware of her surroundings there's a chance he wouldn't have been able to drag her in the first place.

I never understood the "wearing sunglasses at night" trend either, but for obvious lack of visibility and awareness reasons, this is also a "no go." It lessens your overall visibility and peripheral vision (thus lessening your ability to be vigilant), unless you're someone who wears the transition lenses, of course.

## Safety Precautions While Traveling:

**AVOID Rest Stops:**
If driving alone with your kids, avoid rest stops at all costs. Go to regular gas stations, restaurants, etc. I know that rest stops have the best level of accommodations, so I get any apprehension to skip them, but when traveling alone with children especially, it's just not a good idea. Why risk it if you don't have to? Rest stops are very well-known hotbeds for all sorts of crimes, especially prostitution, trafficking, and drug deals.

Also, never leave your kids in the car, even if you have to run in for just a quick second. Sisters and Brothers, it's not worth it. I'll even bring the whole car seat of my sleeping baby inside a gas station to use the restroom. Super, mega, pain in the behind, but so much better than the alternative. The swiftness at which someone could smash out your window and steal your baby is just alarming. You just cannot rely on bystanders to act swiftly nor powerful enough to stop a crime in progress. Plus, it's illegal in several states as well, since there's been a growing rate of incidents of Pediatric Vehicular Stroke (PCS).

**Fueling Up:**
Whenever I'm gassing up my tank, I also grab my keys, wallet, and phone, and lock my children in the car, and DO NOT leave them at all. I always pay at the pump. If I can't pay at the pump, I find another pump!

Keep in mind that key fobs these days can automatically unlock (and in some instances start) a car simply because you are near. So, you need to be attentive.

**Travel Tips:**
- Avoid Rest stops; go to regular gas stations and restaurants instead.
- Rest stops are hotbeds for all sorts of illegal activities.
- Never leave your kids in the car, even for a quick bathroom break.
- When fueling up your gas tank, lock your car, and ensure you have your keys with you.

**Hotels:**
First, whenever we'd check into a hotel room, I always score the place for hidden cameras, something my husband always laughed at me for doing. Could be paranoia or could be too many 20/20 insider scoops about "peeping Tom's." Yall, and my hubby is a well-trained Army Combat Ranger, and he still laughs at me......but, whatever!

Secondly, I always plug up the "peephole" in our hotel room door with tissue paper. I was taught in my years of study that there's a cheap handheld device that almost looks like a magnifying glass, that robbers can use to reverse the function of a peephole, and look in on you or identify if you have expensive items worth stealing. Plugging that hole with tissue paper eliminates that possibility. And when or if you allow the maid to come in and clean, make sure that hole is still plugged up after they leave.

Thirdly, maybe an obvious note to take, but you want to have your doors locked at all times. You don't want to allow your children to walk down to the lobby or to the pool by themselves. When people book hotel rooms, they could very easily leave an anonymous name with the front desk when doing so.

Therefore, if your child was abducted by the "Patron in room 101" it would be very hard to track that person down. You want to be especially cautious of this in more child-friendly family resorts and amusement parks. I hate to break it to you, but places that attract children are going to also attract pedophiles and traffickers. Especially in places where the crowd is always abundant; this makes locating a lost child much more difficult.

In Victimology class, we were taught to choose a room away from an exit; as those rooms are more easily accessed by the outside public, instead of those staying at the hotel. You can always ask the front desk for a hotel map to choose a better room, or you can usually book a room more centrally located ahead of your check-in time.

Lastly, booking an AirBnB or VRBO is actually safer than a hotel. Because patrons have to actually register their real names, addresses, etc., and because you're away from a larger crowd of others.

**Lodging Tips to Remember:**
- Use tissue paper to plug up the door peephole from the inside.
- Keep doors locked at all times, leave the TV on when you leave.
- Don't allow children to walk the halls nor "common areas" of the hotels alone.
- Be aware that people don't actually have to register their real names in order to check into a hotel.

**Public Bathrooms:**

Even if you're a mother of boys or a father of girls, it's better to take your younger child into the bathroom with you, and if you can manage, into the stall with you. You just never know who could snatch your kid coming out of a stall, while you're busy still doing your business.

## Part 3: Education:

Okay, now as promised, let's get into the hard stuff:..

Hard Fact #1:
According to RAINN.com (Rape, Abuse & Incest National Network) of the sexual abuse cases reported to law enforcement, 93% of juvenile victims knew the perpetrator and 59% were acquaintances.

That's just of the crimes that are reported. The most underreported crimes out there, are in fact sex crimes. As in the entire category of sex crimes.

Hard Fact #2:
Young boys are just as much of a target for abduction into the human trafficking world as young girls are; in some cases, little boys are targeted even heavier.

Hard Fact #3:
Everyone thinks, "that could never happen in my neighborhood." But the truth is, ANY CRIME can happen in ANY NEIGHBORHOOD.

Let me give you an example...

I watched a Mel Robbins report on stories from trafficking survivors and one of the women talked about how the teenage boy that lived in the cul-de-sac down the street was trafficking her every time she went to her grandmother's house.

He had lured her into his house because he was a popular kid, and she was a young middle schooler learning about her body, her place in the world, and hadn't yet hit puberty. After a few times of them hanging out, he gained her trust. On one of the occasions she was there, another man was waiting, and this teenage boy sold her into sex slavery that day; that's how she lost her virginity.

I cannot remember if he threatened her life, or the life of her Grandmother if she said anything, but essentially she felt trapped. So, anytime she'd go to her Grandmother's house, which was apparently often, he'd go over, knock on the door, ask the Grandmother if she could come over, and the trafficking would ensue. It was horrifying to hear how this girl felt completely trapped to do anything different, for fear of something happening to her Grandmother or her if she didn't comply.

Hard Fact #4:
People who are abusing children now, don't necessarily have a history of child abuse. It's just a decision. It's just more comfortable to assume, "oh well that person wasn't taught any better." No. Most abusers do NOT have a history of being abused themselves. It is their CHOICE; not necessarily a learned behavior.

Hard Fact #5:
There is no ONE treatment for pedophiles. They are incarcerated if caught, some are then treated while incarcerated.....some are not, and then they're released again. So, we cannot rely on a prison sentence for these criminals to be a deterrent. Speaking strictly as a mother- not as a savant of the Law- there is ZERO punishment harsh enough to justify the crime of hurting a child in this way.

When I look at the average prison sentence of a pedophile, I'm always alarmed at how mild the punishment is.

If the previous fact also angers you, as it does me, it's time we rally our congressman to fund better research on treatment/rehabilitation of pedophiles, and/or harsher sentences such as the death penalty.

Yall- I wrote my senior paper in college on "The Treatment of Pedophiles" back in 2009, and the research I've conducted TODAY still shows zero changes. The fact that there's no one universal treatment for them, outside of mild prison sentences, is alarming to me. Why isn't the death sentence up for grabs on this crime?

Again- not here to argue politics, but I certainly don't want a pedophile out roaming the streets where MY children are, even after he or she has "served their time." Do you? Especially when they're not even treated. They are just locked up and then eventually released.

Something to think about.

**Prevention:**
Now that those hard facts are out of the way, let's take a deep breath and dive into how you can prevent this. And even further, how you could possibly rescue another child (or human being for that matter) out of a potentially harmful environment.

All of this information I'm equipping you with is not to cause paranoia nor anxiety, but to simply equip you. It may feel overwhelming at first, but this is how we as Watchdogs, stand up for our vulnerable. For our tired, weak, weary, and naive. When you picked up this book, you decided you cared enough to do something about this too. You may feel tired and weak now, but with practice, you can be the Hero your circle needs.

Speaking of circle....when it comes to adults you allow them in your "circle," you want to watch how they interact with people they know. And when I say, "circle" I mean anyone you allow to spend any sort of personal time with you and/or your family. This means in your home, alone with your kids, those who teach at your kids' schools, those who lead boy scout groups, those who teach or volunteer at little league, those who are hanging around your neighborhood swimming pool, etc. YOU CHOOSE who is in your circle, and your circle includes your children.

I'm not saying to storm into your child's school and interview everyone in the faculty before you allow your child to attend. But I AM saying, I encourage unannounced drop-ins to school and other activities your child is involved in. I remember once that another mother from school called me and was alarmed to let me know that our children's Christian academy was a registered voting poll for our county and that there was a line out the door of people waiting to get in. Considering this private academy was normally locked uptight, and we had to be buzzed in, this was very alarming to me. I immediately drove down to the school to assess the situation. The staff was not at all taken back by my dropping by; they appreciated my concern. And they were happy to walk me through the precautions they were taking and showed me the security guards standing watch to ensure everyone walked in, voted, and left.

While I trusted the school's precautionary measures, the "what if" still didn't sit right to me. As did not being informed ahead of time. So, I pulled my 4-year-old out of school that day and reported to the other mother what I was doing, so she did the same.

She was a Watchdog for me that day, and I, her. That's how simple it is to step into this role, my friends.

The point being, these are things you want to look out for. If a staff/faculty is unwilling to answer your questions, and not forthcoming about opening up their "usually locked down school" to the public for the day, that's most definitely a red flag.

Observe how potty breaks are handled. How your child's demeanor is before or after school. And make it a habit to ask random questions to your child, to catch them off guard and see how they react. I constantly get on my children's level and will throw them for a loop, to ask if anyone touched their parts. And I watch how they respond. I'll ask how their day was, did anyone new come to class to visit, how they like their teachers, etc.

Not every day, friends. Don't start stressing about having to add yet another thing to your to-do list. Just a new habit for you to begin thinking about and considering, ok?

For as long as I could, I avoided the "how are babies made?" Question. I also avoided the, "how did I get OUT OF your belly?" Question too.

We all have one of those "asks all the questions" children, right?

Well at 5 years old, my child would not let up. I did a poll on Facebook and a majority of my peers felt that woman to woman, explaining our body parts to our little girl was important. So, I did. My 5-year-old doesn't understand sex yet; and gosh, I'm just not ready to explain that.

However, she knows how she was delivered. And what that felt like for momma, and that both she and her sister nursed from my breasts.

Why is this important to explain in regards to "not being a victim?" Because, along with explaining the form and function of our body parts, I was able to elaborate on the sacredness of them, that they are private and a perfect creation by God, and that no one should be asked to, nor trying to touch any part of her body. especially other adults. Because I was willing to give in to her slew of questions, she was in turn more willing to hear me out too. Does that make sense? It was a little give and take.

**Neighborhood Safety:**
You want to teach your kiddos to trust their guts and that if they feel uncomfortable around any adults, they need to voice that no matter what that adult's "position" is in their life.

Also- when you're driving around the neighborhood, it would be good to point out to your kiddos, "that's such and such's house, and that's a safe house. But that blue house there, we don't know them. So we don't go to that house, but we can go to such and such's house for help if we don't feel safe."

For whatever reason too, a crowd responds better to a person yelling, "Fire" or "Rape" versus yelling, "Help."

When in doubt, teach your kid which stores or public places to run to or get to if they're in trouble and need to help. Which phone numbers to dial and who is in their trusted circle.

**Trafficking Education Continued:**

Your teenager has likely already been targeted before. If someone hasn't attempted to get pictures or videos out of them yet, then someone may be trying to get THEM TO BE a trafficker. (Aka someone who does the luring, abducting, or coercing, to get other teens or adolescents into slavery.) Human traffickers aren't always men. Several women are employed by traffickers, to lure other women, teens, and children into "the life."

Trafficking isn't just some random, unorganized crime that has just begun popping up. It is modern-day slavery with tons of research and wildly intelligent tactics, fueling the efficacy of the operation. If you were a teenage girl, and another female peer was painting a picture of a fun, secret, underground life, that includes lots of money, and attention..... you'd likely be curious. You could easily be seduced by the secrecy of it, and that's kind of the appeal around it for teenagers.

The trafficker usually isn't telling these girls, "PS- instead of the money and attention, and excitement you think this is, you're actually going to be raped multiple times a day, by multiple people, and treated like actual garbage while you live in a cage."

There are many tactics and stories told, by peers that lure other peers into these rings. By the time they realize the horrors of what this situation actually is, the trafficker has money in hand, and the victim is now being held against his/her own will.

Most women traffickers are well-trained in psychological warfare and coercion. There are no lengths they'll stop at, to bring more kids in. That, OR they too are being trafficked, and being forced against their will, to pull more kids into the same torture they're receiving on the daily. One simply cannot underestimate the power of drug addiction on these victims as well. More often than not, as soon as a victim is captured, they're immediately pumped full of drugs so that they become reliant on their traffickers to get them their "fix," and thus the victims are weakened in strength and will power for any escape tactics.

It's a horrifying thought imagining a child hooked up to a heroin drip, isn't it? I shudder at the thought. Remember, you cannot discount any lengths that traffickers will go to, to abduct and then secure a human being in this world; it just may be their actual meal ticket.

**Warning signs:**

What most parents don't realize, is that your child and/or YOU, are more likely to be physically harmed or attacked by someone you "know" vs a random attack by a stranger. And this is the threat that is most often overlooked.

Watch how these people interact with kids versus how they interact with adults. If they don't like addressing adults and prefer to address children (think Boy Scout leaders, swim instructors, clergymen, etc) this is a big red flag. Also, any adult with poor social skills, in general, that is around your children a lot, just be wary. This is often a sign that this individual doesn't possess matured social skills, and is thus another factor causing their desire to get closer to children versus adults. This could then fuel one's desire for a relationship with an adolescent rather than an adult.

Crimes of attack on you or on your child aren't really about sex; they're more about power and/or acceptance. And any adult who has a hard time relating to other adults, that can win influence with children easier, is someone of whom you should be wary.

You also want to be aware of adults (that don't have children) who offer to babysit. Most adults don't just suggest that or even adults who have children, who are quick to offer that up when you barely know one another. Who does that, right?

Something else that should tip off all parents, is any adult who is in a position on a field trip, or outing where they are in charge of a lot of kids and refuse help from other adults. RED FLAG. Any adult in their right mind who has to chaperone more than 5 kids on their own would gladly take help! Glaadddddlyyyyyy. That is unless there's a possible ulterior motive for wanting to be alone with a bunch of children.

Places that attract a lot of kids, will also attract a lot of pedophiles and/or human traffickers, so always be vigilant. i.e. family resorts, water parks, parks, schools, churches, arcades, fast food joints with play places, malls, shopping centers, etc.

Pedophiles/traffickers will also try to gain employment in places where they can easily be in charge of a group of adolescents. It's a sad reality, but that's just the truth. Remember, that a lot of them can pass a background check because the sex offender registry only applies to those who have been CAUGHT; cases of sexual assault and pedophilia go unreported every day.

Warning Signs Summary List:
- You're more likely to be targeted by someone you/your family knows than a random act by a stranger.
- Watch how the people in your "inner circle" interact with your kids, and then how they interact with adults. If any of these individuals prefer addressing children over adults, be wary.
- Crimes of attack on children aren't usually about sex; they're often about power.
- Places that attract a lot of kids (such as amusement parks and such) also attract pedophiles and traffickers.
- Sex Offender Registries are only for sex offenders that have been CAUGHT.

## **Who are Likely Targets:**

- Homeless individuals
- Runaways
- Lower economic status individuals
- Those with poor family relationships
- Those who were abused
- Those who were neglected
- Those who feel isolated
- Addicts
- Immigrants

Parents.....that list above? Some of those listed vulnerabilities could easily be your teenager. Isolation, neglect, poor family relationships, or maybe even a lower economic status applies to many families.

Hold up. Before you get mad at me and throw this book out.....this is in no way me calling you a neglectful parent, a poor parent, or a bad parent. Hear me out for a minute.

When you look back on your teenage years, what do you remember about your ATTITUDE? About your FEELINGS? About your OUTLOOK? How about....what were some tough situations you were faced with??

Okay. When you think about those things did those thoughts and instances bring you to a time where you felt really loved and supported by your parents? Or were they thoughts of:

Anarchy! Resistance! I do what I want! No one understands me! That was so stupid and no one listened!

My point being, if we polled a bunch of 30-60-year-olds and asked them if given a chance, would they redo their Teenage years....most of them would quickly reply, "NO." or a "HECKKKKKKK TO THE NO."

Why? Because those years were tough......emotionally, hormonally, and even politically. And not necessarily because of what their parents did or didn't do. It's just because those teenage years bring feelings of NEGLECT, ISOLATION, STRAINED FAMILY RELATIONSHIPS.....for every single teenager. Not one teenager was ever exempt from feeling all 3 of those at one point.

EVEN IF THE ONLY REASON they remember feeling that way, is simply due to the fact that teenage hormones exaggerate and bring drama to evvvveryyyyyything, it. Is. still. A. vulnerability.

Even if they had no just reason for feeling that way, having those feelings is enough to do some crazy things. Perception is everything, my friends. Perception is what causes more people to act before thinking things through. If we counted up all the bone-head things each of us did before thinking, I'm sure we'd have some pretty high numbers to report, yeah? #BeHonest

So, to drive this point home…..you could be THE MOST involved, understanding, and award-winning parent on planet Earth, and your child still can or already has felt all three emotions. It's just par for the course in those teenage angst years.

Therefore, your teenage child, with these vulnerabilities, is susceptible to being a target, and that is not a point to sleep on. For teenagers specifically, a big way they are targeted is through their devices. But if you have children using devices at all, no matter their age, this is a channel through which they could be targeted. And they'll be targeted….relentlessly, to no end, so this is where education becomes power.

## Social Media, The Internet, and Gaming Devices:

I think we can all agree that information regarding safeguarding our children in these instances, has become more abundant, and for that I am grateful. However, as stated previously.... Crime intelligence is ever-evolving constantly, and a safeguard that was previously impenetrable may now be weakened. So my best suggestion is this:

1) If your child is old enough to have any sort of social media account, you definitely want to have a conversation with them about keeping their profiles locked down and private, to only friends they know in person. AT LEAST until they are 18 or older. And regularly check their app usage to ensure there isn't an app unknown to you. I've heard GREAT THINGS about the "Bark app" which safeguards your teen's/adolescents from inappropriate messaging and will alert you as soon as one is detected.

2) Check your child's text messages, DM's, Instant Messages, emails, etc, regularly. Not to invade their privacy, or with the intent of making them feel like you don't trust them, but to stress that you don't trust others.

3) If your children are young like mine, you can choose to absolve the issue in its entirety, and not allow access to social media, games, etc. You can also just simply ensure there are child locks and/or very secure parental guidance apps on there. My children are not able to write and read yet, so I'm not super worried. But, I do regularly pop in and watch the youtube videos that they're watching on "kids youtube" just to ensure the movies or story scenarios aren't inappropriate nor set up for grooming.

4) If your child is a gamer with a headset where they can regularly chat online, ensure ZERO personal information is discussed; that they're only discussing the game. And if at all possible, you want to look into putting a safeguard on this as well. I don't know a whole lot about gaming, admittedly, but my understanding is that you can create a profile claiming to be any age, and there are no regulations in place to validate that or not. So, you just want to have that talk with your kiddos, and regularly check in on those conversations during game times. Even just set specific game times, when you can be present to check-in or hide the game counsel away during the times you're not available. It's really up to you and your parenting style and the level of understanding your kid has for the severity of this topic. Trust your gut.

5) If you notice your child, or an acquaintance of your child posting expensive items on social media suddenly, or being more secretive, or suddenly acting or dressing more sexualized, speak up and get involved. This could be linked to being solicited on the internet, or someone perhaps sending them gifts in exchange for pornographic content. Any messages your child is receiving saying, how mature they are for their age, and how they're so pretty they could be a model, that is Grooming 101.

**Identifying Victims:**
There are physical, emotional, and behavioral Signs. The physical signs maybe a little more obvious, but here are some to look for.

**Physical signs:**
Evidence of violence such as broken bones, STDs, concussions, burn marks, bruising, cuts, or signs of restraint or torture. Also, two or more people gathered in the same location with the exact same tattoo or branding mark in the exact same spot; often traffickers brand their people like cattle.

You also want to pay attention to the appearance of someone not fitting the setting. Example: A really nicely dressed male in a suit and tie, walking around with a dirty-looking younger boy, whose eyes are downcast, clothing is ragged, and he's looking to the older gentlemen before speaking.

**Emotional Signs:**
These range all over the place, and could easily just be chalked up to the mood swings of a hormonal teenager. So dig in deeper before assuming that is the case.

Some of them are:
Depression, fear, PTSD, hopelessness, helplessness, anxiety, suicidal thoughts, or actions, poor posture, allowing someone else to speak, resistance to authority or 1st responders, paranoia, and often may not identify as a victim.

**Behavioral Signs:**
There may be an influx of new slang usage or inappropriate behavior, or they may be suddenly accompanied by an older individual. They could be withdrawn, unusually tired, have major swings in mood and uncharacteristic behaviors, or bragging about new money, modeling, or a new boyfriend/girlfriend.

## Conclusion:

There you have it, Parents. I have dumped out every bit of information I have on this topic, how to prevent it, and what signs to look for. Though it may feel like an overwhelming amount of information, I knew I wouldn't be able to sleep at night, knowing I had left anything out.

Read it, apply it, and read it again. In fact, I hope you read this book as many times as you need to until you absorb it, and then my intention is that you pass this book down to someone you care about, who may need it. I wanted all my years of education to be summed up in this book for you, in a swift manner, so that you could begin implementing and utilizing it right away.

Time is the most precious commodity we have, and I don't want any more of yours wasted on worrying whether or not you're properly equipped to handle most parents' biggest fears coming true.

On that note, If you'd like to take this thing a little farther, and learn some great physical defense movements or take a course on "Human Trafficking," I'll list some of my favorite sources on my website, www.whitneycarrion.com.

Remember, "Watchdogs possess all the abilities and characteristics of the wolf, with one exception: how they use those abilities. Wolves use their skills in pursuit of evil, while watchdogs protect and defend others.

Watchdogs possess the ability to put aside what they want in the service and defense of others. It's the military people defending the country, the firemen rushing into danger while everyone else runs away, the policeman engaging violent scum so others can sleep safely at night." -dyeager.org

As someone who is reading this book, I hope you have decided to be a Watchdog for your family and others. When the time comes, you will be ready, Good and Faithful Servant.

**I'm praying for you.**

**Acknowledgments:**

Before writing this Parent's Manual, I called my former Victimology Professor, whom I reference many times in this book. Jeanie Thies was one of the coolest Professors from my years of Study at Lindenwood University, in St. Charles, MO. I owe her deep credit for starting this spark of passion for serving my community in this way. Though I was the kid who was always late to her 8 am classes- and that probably made her view me as a disrespectful turd- everything she taught, stuck with me in a deep way. I had no idea it would have such a profound effect on me, causing me to use her teachings in my daily life, and then cause me to write these books nearly 13 years later.

Jeanie, thank you for the work you did to serve me so well back in the day and for continuing to care, teach, and properly educate those who've since come after me. I know that being an educator is one of the most thankless jobs there is, and I'll never understand that. But I assure you that YOU, MA'AM, are making a grave difference today; my hope is that these books impact generations to come. Thank you for helping me do that.

## Jeanie Thies Biography:

Jeanie Thies has been a member of the Lindenwood University (LU) faculty since 2007. She has taught courses in Public Administration, Political Science, and Criminal Justice, and has served as Chair of the MPA program and Dean of Institutional Research. She holds a Ph.D. in Political Science from the University of Missouri-St. Louis, with an emphasis on crime control policy analysis. She also has a master's degree in Psychology from the University of Missouri-St. Louis, and a bachelor's degree in Psychology from the University of Missouri-Columbia. She has over 30 years of experience in the field of criminal justice, including work as a prison psychologist and a program administrator for Missouri's Department of Corrections, and in the areas of training, policy development, and program evaluation for national, state, and local agencies. She has published articles and conducted training on topics such as sex offenders, corrections programming, high-risk youth, treatment courts, and family violence. She is currently a member of the Missouri State Child Abuse and Neglect Review Board and the St. Louis chapter of the Midwestern Innocence Project.

....and let's also not forget, life-changer!

## Acknowledgments Cont'd:

I must also take the time to recognize the incredible crew, who helped me bring these ideas to life. The "Beautifully Designed for More" duo of sisters, Ashley Loveday Shepherd and Keeli Loveday Boyce, took my chaotic idea and helped me streamline it into something that made sense to my ideal consumer. They listened to me vent, dream, jump for joy, panic, and everything in between, and helped my stubborn behind, make this baby mine.

They enlisted the brilliant wisdom of Aimee Larsen in all editing and creative ideas, and Morgan Meschede with Wavelet Designs is who drew and re-drew and re-sized Ronnie the Rhino, over and over, until he matched the idea in my head, better than I had ever dreamed.

All of these women made my labor of love, a labor of their own, and I wouldn't have been able to do this without them.

## About the Author

I am an Army Wife, Mother of 2 Girls, and what you would call a Passionate "Multipreneur." I run one large Social Marketing business, and within one year of doing that, decided to start up a Non-Profit Organization to advocate for Human Trafficking Victims in South Africa, and with that came the vision to write children's books & parents' manual on the same topic. I am an 11 year Professional in the Health and Fitness Industry, and a 3x Gym Owner. So, I now help the burnt-out Fit Pro take their businesses from offline to online, with proven Social Media Strategies that win. I'm also a multi-stage-speaker because the Lord saw it fit to bless me as a visionary. Yes, I'm a follower of Jesus, but I'm from the South-side of the Kingdom; that means to pray with me, don't play with me.

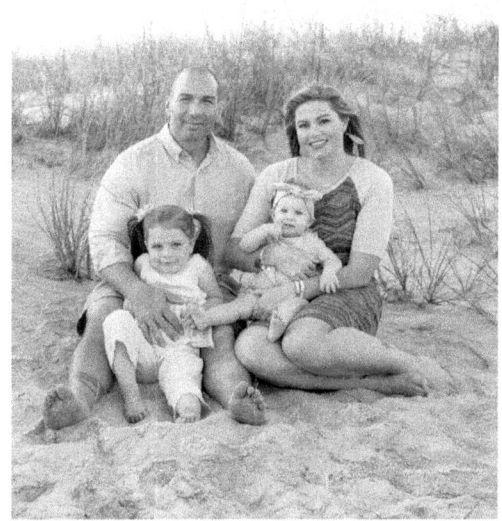

My heart is on fire for serving the Lord and my Country, and helping others step into the truth of whom they were created to be, both selflessly and selfishly. Which is exactly how my multipreneurship came about! When I see a need, and a way to elevate a system or process, I use all my ability to create a system to fill it or pass the idea onto someone else equipped to do so. Part of being a leader, I've always felt, is willing to go first; someone always has to go first and lead the way. And for some reason, I've never been afraid to be the one to take that first step, even if it meant falling on my face in front of others. Some call what I do "taking big risks" or " shooting from the hip," but I call it, "taking leaps of Faith" and "listening to prompts from the Lord."

I fully believe that our steps will not be blessed until we jump ALL IN and that over-thinking is probably getting you underpaid.

So with that- I welcome you to visit my website at www.whitneycarrion.com, and to all the projects that are true labors of love, from each season I birthed them in.

www.ingramcontent.com/pod-product-compliance
Lightning Source LLC
Chambersburg PA
CBHW071126030426
42336CB00013BA/2217